RENAL DIET COOKBOOK FOR VEGANS

Understanding Kidney Disease, and Using Delicious Varieties of Plant-Based Recipes for Prevention

Jeremy Owen

Contents

Introduction

Types and Stages of Kidney Disease

The Role of Diet in Kidney Health

Why a Vegan Diet?

Essential Nutrients for Kidney Health

Breakfast Recipes

Lunch Recipes

Dinner Recipes

Desserts

Kidney-Friendly Sweet Treats

Hydration Tips for Kidney Health

Meal Planning and Preparation

Conclusion

Introduction

Hello there! I'm glad you're here, taking the time to understand kidney disease. Whether you're reading this because you or someone close to you is dealing with kidney issues, or you just want to be proactive about your health, you're making a fantastic choice. Knowledge is power, and understanding how our bodies work, especially the crucial role our kidneys play, can be incredibly empowering. Before we go into other businesses featured in this Cookbook, Let's look into this topic together, step by step, and uncover what kidney disease is all about, why it matters, and what you can do to support kidney health.

Let me paint a picture of the kidneys. They're these two bean-shaped organs located just below your ribcage, one on each side of your spine. Despite their modest size, they're powerhouse organs. Their primary job is to filter your blood, removing waste products and excess substances to create urine. They also balance your body's fluids, regulate blood pressure, produce certain hormones, and help keep your bones strong by managing calcium and phosphorus levels. Imagine them as the diligent housekeepers of your body, keeping everything in order.

Now, when we talk about kidney disease, we're referring to conditions that damage your kidneys and decrease their ability to keep your body clean and chemically balanced. Kidney disease can be acute (sudden) or chronic (long-term). Chronic kidney disease (CKD) is the most common form, and it usually progresses slowly over time. According to the National Kidney Foundation, CKD affects over 10% of the global population. That's a significant number, and what's even more concerning is that many people with CKD are unaware they have it because the early stages often present no symptoms.

So, why should you care about your kidneys? Well, when kidneys are damaged, waste products and fluids can build up in the body, causing swelling in your ankles, vomiting, weakness, poor sleep, and shortness of breath. If left untreated, kidney disease can lead to serious complications, including heart disease, nerve damage, and weak bones. In the advanced stages, kidney disease can lead to kidney failure, at which point dialysis or a kidney transplant is necessary to sustain life.

It's clear that keeping your kidneys healthy is vital, but how do we do that? This is where diet and lifestyle come into play, especially the benefits of a vegan diet in managing and preventing kidney disease. Let's explore this further with some scientific backing.

Research has shown that diet plays a crucial role in kidney health. A study published in the Clinical Journal of the American Society of Nephrology found that plant-based diets are associated with a lower risk of kidney disease progression. One reason for this is that plant-based diets are naturally lower in protein compared to animal-based diets. High protein intake, especially from animal sources, can increase the workload on the kidneys. When your kidneys are already compromised, the last thing they need is extra stress. By choosing plant-based proteins like beans, lentils, tofu, and quinoa, you're giving your kidneys a much-needed break.

Moreover, plant-based diets are rich in antioxidants and anti-inflammatory compounds. Chronic inflammation and oxidative stress are key players in the progression of kidney disease. Fruits, vegetables, whole grains, nuts, and seeds are packed with antioxidants that help neutralize harmful free radicals and reduce inflammation. For instance, berries are known for their high antioxidant content. Including them in your diet can provide protective benefits for your kidneys.

Another important factor to consider is the intake of minerals like potassium and phosphorus. These are essential for your health, but when your kidneys aren't functioning properly, they can build up in your body. High potassium levels can cause heart problems, while excess phosphorus can lead to bone and heart issues. Many plant-based foods are naturally lower in these minerals compared to animal-based foods. For example, while bananas are high in potassium, apples, berries, and carrots are excellent lower-potassium alternatives.

Staying hydrated is another crucial aspect of kidney health. Water helps your kidneys remove waste from your blood in the form of urine. It also helps keep your blood vessels open so that blood can move freely to your kidneys and deliver essential nutrients to them. However, it's important to balance your fluid intake, especially if your kidneys are already damaged. Drinking too much or too little can strain them further. Aim to drink water when you're thirsty and monitor your intake based on your doctor's advice.

Now, let's talk about sodium. High sodium intake is linked to increased blood pressure, which is a major risk factor for kidney disease. Processed foods are often high in sodium, so one of the best things you can do for your kidneys is to reduce your intake of these foods. Instead, flavor your meals with herbs, spices, and natural flavorings like lemon juice or vinegar. These not only enhance the taste of your food but also offer additional health benefits.

Incorporating a vegan diet isn't just about avoiding animal products; it's about embracing a variety of nutrient-dense, plant-based foods that support overall health. For those with kidney disease, it's essential to work with a dietitian to ensure you're meeting your nutritional needs while managing your condition. They can help you tailor a diet plan that suits your individual health status and lifestyle.

Another critical aspect of managing kidney disease is regular medical checkups. Early detection and treatment can slow the progression of kidney disease. Regular blood and urine tests can help monitor kidney function and detect any abnormalities early on. If you have risk factors for kidney disease, such as diabetes, high blood pressure, or a family history of kidney problems, it's even more important to stay on top of these screenings.

Let's not forget the impact of lifestyle choices beyond diet. Physical activity, maintaining a healthy weight, and avoiding smoking can all contribute to better kidney health. Exercise helps control blood pressure and blood sugar levels, both of which are crucial for preventing kidney damage. Aim for at least 30 minutes of moderate exercise most days of the week. This could be as simple as a brisk walk, cycling, or even gardening.

Stress management is another often-overlooked aspect of kidney health. Chronic stress can contribute to high blood pressure and other harmful behaviors like poor eating habits or smoking. Practices like meditation, deep breathing exercises, and yoga can help manage stress levels and improve overall well-being.

In conclusion, understanding kidney disease and taking steps to manage it through diet and lifestyle changes can make a significant difference in your health and quality of life. Embracing a vegan diet rich in plant-based foods, staying hydrated, reducing sodium intake, and maintaining a healthy lifestyle are all powerful tools in supporting your kidneys. Remember, it's about making informed choices that align with your health needs and working closely with healthcare professionals to monitor and manage your condition. Your kidneys are vital organs that deserve the best care, and with the right approach, you can take charge of your kidney health and live a full, healthy life.

Types and Stages of Kidney Disease

Kidney disease can be broadly classified into two main types: Acute Kidney Injury (AKI) and Chronic Kidney Disease (CKD). Understanding these types and their stages is crucial for effective management and treatment.

Acute Kidney Injury (AKI): AKI, previously known as acute renal failure, is a sudden and often temporary loss of kidney function. It can develop over a few hours or days and is typically the result of an event that causes severe damage to the kidneys. Common causes of AKI include severe dehydration, a sudden drop in blood flow to the kidneys due to injury or surgery, exposure to certain toxins, or complications from medications. The hallmark of AKI is its rapid onset, which can lead to an accumulation of waste products in the blood, imbalance in electrolytes, and fluid overload. Prompt medical intervention is crucial to address the underlying cause and support kidney recovery.

Chronic Kidney Disease (CKD): CKD is a long-term condition characterized by the gradual loss of kidney function over time. It is usually irreversible and can progress to end-stage renal disease (ESRD) if not managed effectively. CKD is commonly caused by conditions such as diabetes, hypertension, chronic glomerulonephritis (inflammation of the kidney's filtering units), and polycystic kidney disease (a genetic disorder). Unlike AKI, CKD progresses slowly and often silently, with symptoms becoming apparent only in the later stages.

CKD is categorized into five stages based on the glomerular filtration rate (GFR), which measures how well the kidneys filter blood:

- Stage 1 (GFR ≥ 90 mL/min): In this stage, the kidneys function normally, but there may be structural abnormalities or evidence of kidney damage, such as protein in the urine. Most people are asymptomatic and often unaware they have CKD.

- Stage 2 (GFR 60-89 mL/min): There is a mild reduction in kidney function. Like Stage 1, symptoms are usually absent, but monitoring and lifestyle changes are essential to prevent progression.

- Stage 3 (GFR 30-59 mL/min): This stage is divided into 3a (GFR 45-59 mL/min) and 3b (GFR 30-44 mL/min). Moderate reduction in kidney function is present, and symptoms such as fatigue, swelling, and changes in urination may begin to appear. This is a critical stage for intervention to slow further decline.

- Stage 4 (GFR 15-29 mL/min): Severe reduction in kidney function occurs in this stage. Symptoms become more pronounced, including significant fatigue, swelling, anemia, and bone disease. Preparation for potential dialysis or kidney transplant should begin.

- Stage 5 (GFR < 15 mL/min): Also known as end-stage renal disease (ESRD), at this stage, kidney function is minimal, and dialysis or a kidney transplant is required to sustain life. Symptoms are severe and can include nausea, vomiting, difficulty breathing, and cognitive impairment.

Understanding these stages helps in tailoring treatment and management strategies to slow progression and improve quality of life for individuals with CKD.

The Role of Diet in Kidney Health

Diet plays an essential role in maintaining kidney health and managing kidney disease. The kidneys are responsible for filtering waste products from the blood, balancing electrolytes, and regulating fluid levels. What we eat can significantly impact these processes and either support or burden kidney function.

Protein Intake: One of the critical dietary considerations for kidney health is protein intake. The kidneys process the waste products of protein metabolism, and excessive protein can increase the workload on the kidneys.

While protein is essential for overall health, moderation is key, especially for those with kidney disease. Plant-based proteins, such as beans, lentils, tofu, and quinoa, are recommended over animal-based proteins because they generate fewer waste products and are generally easier for the kidneys to handle.

Phosphorus and Potassium Management: Phosphorus and potassium are minerals that play vital roles in the body but can be problematic when kidney function is compromised. Healthy kidneys maintain the balance of these minerals, but in kidney disease, they can accumulate to dangerous levels. High phosphorus levels can lead to bone disease and cardiovascular issues, while elevated potassium levels can cause severe heart problems. Dietary adjustments are necessary to manage these minerals. Foods low in phosphorus include fresh fruits and vegetables, while high-potassium foods like bananas, oranges, and potatoes should be limited or substituted with lower-potassium options such as apples, berries, and carrots.

Sodium Reduction: Sodium is another crucial factor in kidney health. High sodium intake can increase blood pressure and worsen kidney damage. Reducing sodium helps manage blood pressure and reduces fluid buildup, which is beneficial for kidney health. Avoiding processed foods, using herbs and spices for flavor, and cooking at home can help control sodium intake.

Hydration: Adequate hydration is essential for kidney function, as it helps flush out toxins and waste products from the blood. However, the amount of fluid intake should be balanced, particularly in advanced kidney disease, where fluid restriction might be necessary. Drinking water throughout the day and monitoring fluid intake based on medical advice is important for maintaining kidney health.

Antioxidants and Anti-inflammatory Foods: A diet rich in antioxidants and anti-inflammatory foods can protect the kidneys from oxidative stress and inflammation, both of which contribute to kidney damage. Fruits, vegetables, nuts, seeds, and whole grains are excellent sources of antioxidants. Berries, for example, are particularly high in antioxidants and have been shown to provide protective benefits for the kidneys.

Whole Grains and Fiber: Whole grains and high-fiber foods support kidney health by promoting better blood sugar control and reducing the risk of diabetes, a major risk factor for kidney disease. Foods like oatmeal, brown rice, whole wheat, and barley are nutritious options that can be included in a kidney-friendly diet.

Healthy Fats: Including healthy fats in the diet, such as those found in avocados, nuts, seeds, and olive oil, is beneficial for overall health and can support kidney function by reducing inflammation and promoting cardiovascular health.

Calcium and Vitamin D: Maintaining adequate levels of calcium and vitamin D is important for bone health, which can be compromised in kidney disease. Calcium-rich foods like fortified plant milks and leafy greens, along with adequate sunlight exposure or supplementation for vitamin D, are important for maintaining bone strength.

In summary, a balanced diet that includes a variety of nutrient-dense, plant-based foods, while managing protein, sodium, phosphorus, and potassium intake, can significantly support kidney health and help manage kidney disease.

Why a Vegan Diet?

Adopting a vegan diet can offer numerous benefits for kidney health, particularly for those managing kidney disease. A vegan diet excludes all animal products, including meat, dairy, and eggs, focusing instead on plant-based foods such as fruits, vegetables, grains, nuts, and seeds. There are several compelling reasons why a vegan diet is beneficial for kidney health.

Lower Protein Load: One of the primary advantages of a vegan diet is the lower protein load compared to animal-based diets. While protein is necessary for the body, excessive protein intake can strain the kidneys, especially when the protein comes from animal sources. Plant-based proteins are easier on the kidneys and produce fewer waste products. This can help reduce the workload on the kidneys and slow the progression of kidney disease.

Reduced Risk of Diabetes and Hypertension: Diabetes and hypertension are the leading causes of CKD. A vegan diet, rich in fiber, antioxidants, and low in saturated fats, helps manage blood sugar levels and blood pressure. Whole grains, legumes, fruits, and vegetables promote better blood sugar control and reduce insulin resistance, lowering the risk of diabetes. Additionally, the high fiber content in plant-based foods helps regulate blood pressure, which is crucial for kidney health.

Lower Phosphorus Intake: Animal-based foods are high in phosphorus, which can be problematic for those with kidney disease. Excess phosphorus can lead to bone and heart problems. Plant-based foods generally contain lower levels of phosphorus, and the phosphorus in these foods is less readily absorbed by the body. This helps maintain healthier phosphorus levels and supports overall kidney health.

Antioxidant and Anti-inflammatory Properties: A vegan diet is naturally rich in antioxidants and anti-inflammatory compounds. Chronic inflammation and oxidative stress are significant contributors to kidney damage. By consuming a variety of fruits, vegetables, nuts, seeds, and whole grains, you provide your body with powerful antioxidants that neutralize harmful free radicals and reduce inflammation. This protective effect can slow the progression of kidney disease and improve overall health.

Heart Health: Cardiovascular health is closely linked to kidney health. Heart disease is common in individuals with kidney disease, and a vegan diet supports heart health by lowering cholesterol levels, reducing blood pressure, and improving blood vessel function. Plant-based diets are low in saturated fats and cholesterol, which are prevalent in animal products. Instead, they are rich in heart-healthy fats from sources like avocados, nuts, and seeds.

Weight Management: Maintaining a healthy weight is crucial for managing kidney disease. Obesity increases the risk of developing diabetes and hypertension, both of which are detrimental to kidney health. A vegan diet, which is typically lower in calories and higher in fiber, can help with weight management. The high fiber content of plant-based foods promotes satiety, reducing overall calorie intake and supporting a healthy weight.

Digestive Health: Fiber-rich plant foods support digestive health by promoting regular bowel movements and a healthy gut microbiome. A healthy digestive system is essential for nutrient absorption and overall well-being.

Improved digestion can also reduce the burden on the kidneys, as a healthy gut helps process waste more efficiently.

Ethical and Environmental Benefits: Beyond health benefits, adopting the act of a vegan diet has ethical and environmental advantages. Reducing or eliminating animal products from your diet helps decrease animal suffering and contributes to more sustainable food production practices. Environmental sustainability is increasingly important as climate change and resource depletion become pressing global issues. By choosing plant-based foods, you contribute to a more sustainable future while also taking care of your health.

Essential Nutrients for Kidney Health

Maintaining kidney health involves understanding how different nutrients impact these vital organs. The kidneys filter waste, balance electrolytes, and regulate fluid levels in our bodies. Four key nutrients—protein, phosphorus, potassium, and sodium—play significant roles in kidney function and overall health. Let's dive into each of these nutrients, how they function in the body, and their implications for kidney health.

Protein

Protein is a fundamental building block of the body, essential for the growth, repair, and maintenance of tissues. It plays a crucial role in building muscles, repairing tissues, and producing enzymes and hormones. Proteins are made up of amino acids, which are necessary for various bodily functions, including immune response and energy production.

However, when it comes to kidney health, the type and amount of protein you consume can have significant implications. The kidneys are responsible for filtering waste products generated from protein metabolism. These waste products include urea and creatinine, which need to be efficiently removed from the bloodstream to prevent toxicity.

Why Protein Matters for Kidney Health:
For people with healthy kidneys, consuming a balanced amount of protein is essential for overall health. However, in individuals with kidney disease, particularly chronic kidney disease (CKD), excessive protein intake

can place additional strain on the kidneys. The kidneys have to work harder to eliminate the byproducts of protein metabolism, which can accelerate the progression of kidney damage.

Animal vs. Plant-Based Proteins:
Animal proteins, such as those from meat, poultry, fish, eggs, and dairy products, are complete proteins, meaning they contain all essential amino acids. However, they also generate more waste products compared to plant-based proteins. On the other hand, plant-based proteins, found in beans, lentils, tofu, tempeh, nuts, and seeds, produce fewer waste products and are generally easier for the kidneys to process. While plant proteins may not always be complete on their own, combining different plant sources can provide all essential amino acids.

Moderation is Key:

For individuals with CKD, moderating protein intake is crucial. According to the National Kidney Foundation, a controlled protein intake can help slow the progression of kidney disease and reduce the risk of complications. It's often recommended to consult with a healthcare professional or dietitian to determine the appropriate amount of protein based on the stage of kidney disease and individual health needs.

In Summary:
Protein is vital for overall health, but its management is crucial for those with kidney concerns. Opting for plant-based proteins and moderating total protein intake can help support kidney function and slow disease progression.

Phosphorus

Phosphorus is a mineral that plays a vital role in the formation of bones and teeth, energy production, and the regulation of muscle and nerve function. It is found in many foods, including dairy products, meat, fish, poultry, nuts, beans, and whole grains. Phosphorus works in tandem with calcium to maintain bone health and cellular function.

Why Phosphorus Matters for Kidney Health:
Healthy kidneys regulate phosphorus levels in the blood by excreting excess amounts through urine. However, in individuals with kidney disease, the kidneys' ability to remove excess phosphorus diminishes. High levels of phosphorus in the blood can lead to hyperphosphatemia, which can cause serious complications such as bone and cardiovascular diseases.

Phosphorus and Bone Health:

Excessive phosphorus levels can pull calcium out of the bones, making them weak and brittle, a condition known as renal osteodystrophy. High phosphorus can also lead to the calcification of blood vessels and organs, increasing the risk of heart disease.

Managing Phosphorus Intake:
For those with CKD, it is crucial to manage phosphorus intake to prevent these complications. Limiting foods high in phosphorus, such as dairy products, processed foods, and colas, can help maintain balanced levels. Additionally, some plant-based foods contain phosphorus in a form called phytate, which is less absorbable by the human body, making plant-based diets beneficial in managing phosphorus levels.

Phosphate Binders:
In some cases, doctors may prescribe phosphate binders, medications that

help prevent the absorption of phosphorus from the foods consumed. These are taken with meals and can be effective in controlling phosphorus levels in the blood.

In Summary:
Phosphorus is essential for bone health and energy production, but managing its intake is crucial for individuals with kidney disease. Opting for plant-based sources and, when necessary, using phosphate binders can help control phosphorus levels and prevent complications.

Potassium

Potassium is an essential mineral and electrolyte that helps regulate fluid balance, muscle contractions, and nerve signals. It is vital for maintaining normal heart function and muscle contraction. Potassium is found in a variety of foods, including fruits (bananas, oranges), vegetables (potatoes, spinach), and legumes.

Why Potassium Matters for Kidney Health:
The kidneys help maintain the proper balance of potassium in the blood. They filter out excess potassium and excrete it through urine. However, when kidney function declines, the ability to remove excess potassium is impaired, leading to hyperkalemia (high potassium levels). Hyperkalemia can cause dangerous heart rhythms and muscle weakness.

Balancing Potassium Intake:
For individuals with kidney disease, managing potassium intake is essential. While potassium is vital for health, too much can be harmful. Monitoring dietary intake and opting for low-potassium foods can help prevent hyperkalemia. Low-potassium food

choices include apples, berries, carrots, and green beans.

Potassium Binders:
In some cases, healthcare providers may recommend potassium binders, medications that help the body remove excess potassium through the gastrointestinal tract. These are typically used in conjunction with dietary modifications to keep potassium levels within a safe range.

Potassium and Dialysis:
For those undergoing dialysis, managing potassium intake is even more critical, as dialysis can only remove a certain amount of potassium from the blood. Regular monitoring of blood potassium levels and adhering to dietary recommendations are essential for preventing complications.

In Summary:

Potassium is crucial for maintaining fluid balance and proper muscle function, but managing its levels is vital for those with kidney disease. Opting for low-potassium foods and, if necessary, using potassium binders can help maintain safe potassium levels.

Sodium

Sodium is an essential electrolyte that plays a significant role in maintaining fluid balance, nerve function, and muscle contractions. It is commonly found in table salt and many processed foods. Sodium helps regulate blood pressure and volume, ensuring that bodily functions operate smoothly.

Why Sodium Matters for Kidney Health: The kidneys regulate sodium balance by filtering and excreting excess sodium through urine. High sodium intake can lead to fluid retention, increased blood pressure, and edema (swelling). For individuals with kidney disease, managing sodium intake is critical, as the kidneys' ability to excrete sodium is compromised.

Sodium and Blood Pressure:
High sodium intake is directly linked to hypertension (high blood pressure), which is a leading cause of CKD and can worsen existing kidney conditions. Elevated blood pressure can damage the blood vessels in the kidneys, reducing their ability to function properly and leading to further kidney damage.

Reducing Sodium Intake:
For kidney health, it's crucial to limit sodium intake. This can be achieved by avoiding processed foods, which are often high in sodium, and opting for fresh, whole foods instead. Cooking at home and using herbs and spices for flavor instead of salt can also help

reduce sodium consumption. The American Heart Association recommends limiting sodium intake to no more than 2,300 milligrams per day, with an ideal limit of 1,500 milligrams for most adults, especially those with high blood pressure or kidney disease.

Reading Labels:
Becoming a savvy label reader can help you identify high-sodium foods and make healthier choices. Foods labeled as "low sodium" or "no salt added" can be beneficial. Additionally, be cautious of hidden sodium in condiments, sauces, and restaurant meals.

In Summary:
Sodium is essential for fluid balance and nerve function, but managing its intake is vital for maintaining healthy blood pressure and preventing further kidney damage in those with kidney disease. Opting for low-sodium foods and

cooking with fresh ingredients can help control sodium levels.

Breakfast Recipes

Smoothies and Shakes

Berry-Spinach Smoothie
1. Classic Berry-Spinach Smoothie
 - Ingredients: 1 cup fresh or frozen mixed berries, 1 handful fresh spinach, 1 banana, 1 cup almond milk, 1 tablespoon chia seeds.
 - Instructions:
   1. Combine all ingredients in a blender.
   2. Blend until smooth and creamy.
   3. Pour into a glass and serve immediately.

2. Tropical Berry-Spinach Smoothie
 - Ingredients: 1 cup pineapple chunks, 1/2 cup strawberries, 1 handful fresh spinach, 1/2 cup coconut water, 1 tablespoon flaxseeds.
 - Instructions:
   1. Place all ingredients in a blender.

2. Blend on high until fully combined and smooth.
3. Serve in a chilled glass.

3. Protein-Packed Berry-Spinach Smoothie
- Ingredients: 1 cup mixed berries, 1 handful spinach, 1 scoop vegan protein powder, 1 cup oat milk, 1 tablespoon almond butter.
- Instructions:
1. Add all ingredients to a blender.
2. Blend until smooth and no chunks remain.
3. Pour into a glass and enjoy.

4. Green Berry-Spinach Smoothie
- Ingredients: 1 cup blueberries, 1 handful spinach, 1/2 avocado, 1 cup green tea, 1 teaspoon spirulina powder.
- Instructions:
1. Combine all ingredients in a blender.
2. Blend until smooth and well mixed.

3. Serve immediately for the best taste.

Almond Butter Banana Shake
1. Classic Almond Butter Banana Shake
   - Ingredients: 2 bananas, 2 tablespoons almond butter, 1 cup almond milk, 1 teaspoon vanilla extract, 1 tablespoon maple syrup.
   - Instructions:
     1. Add all ingredients to a blender.
     2. Blend until smooth and creamy.
     3. Serve in a tall glass.

2. Chocolate Almond Butter Banana Shake
   - Ingredients: 2 bananas, 2 tablespoons almond butter, 1 cup almond milk, 1 tablespoon cocoa powder, 1 teaspoon vanilla extract.
   - Instructions:
     1. Combine all ingredients in a blender.
     2. Blend until well mixed and smooth.
     3. Pour into a glass and serve.

3. Berry Almond Butter Banana Shake
   - Ingredients: 1 banana, 1/2 cup mixed berries, 2 tablespoons almond butter, 1 cup almond milk, 1 tablespoon chia seeds.
   - Instructions:
     1. Place all ingredients in a blender.
     2. Blend until smooth and creamy.
     3. Serve immediately.

4. Green Almond Butter Banana Shake
   - Ingredients: 1 banana, 1 handful spinach, 2 tablespoons almond butter, 1 cup coconut milk, 1 tablespoon hemp seeds.
   - Instructions:
     1. Combine all ingredients in a blender.
     2. Blend until smooth and well combined.
     3. Serve in a chilled glass.

Breakfast Bowls

Quinoa Porridge with Berries

1. Classic Quinoa Porridge with Berries
   - Ingredients: 1 cup cooked quinoa, 1 cup almond milk, 1 tablespoon maple syrup, 1/2 teaspoon cinnamon, 1 cup mixed berries.
   - Instructions:
     1. In a saucepan, combine cooked quinoa and almond milk.
     2. Heat over medium heat until warm, stirring occasionally.
     3. Stir in maple syrup and cinnamon.
     4. Serve in a bowl topped with mixed berries.

2. Tropical Quinoa Porridge with Berries
   - Ingredients: 1 cup cooked quinoa, 1 cup coconut milk, 1 tablespoon agave syrup, 1/2 teaspoon nutmeg, 1 cup chopped pineapple, 1/2 cup blueberries.
   - Instructions:
     1. Combine cooked quinoa and coconut milk in a saucepan.
     2. Heat over medium heat until warmed through.

3. Stir in agave syrup and nutmeg.

4. Serve in a bowl topped with pineapple and blueberries.

3. Chocolate Quinoa Porridge with Berries

- Ingredients: 1 cup cooked quinoa, 1 cup almond milk, 1 tablespoon cocoa powder, 1 tablespoon maple syrup, 1 cup strawberries.

- Instructions:

1. In a saucepan, combine cooked quinoa, almond milk, and cocoa powder.

2. Heat over medium heat until warmed, stirring to dissolve the cocoa.

3. Stir in maple syrup.

4. Serve in a bowl topped with strawberries.

4. Nutty Quinoa Porridge with Berries

- Ingredients: 1 cup cooked quinoa, 1 cup almond milk, 1 tablespoon almond butter, 1 tablespoon honey, 1 cup raspberries.

- Instructions:

1. Combine cooked quinoa and almond milk in a saucepan.
2. Heat over medium heat until warm.
3. Stir in almond butter and honey until well mixed.
4. Serve in a bowl topped with raspberries.

Tofu Scramble with Veggies
1. Classic Tofu Scramble with Veggies
 - Ingredients: 1 block firm tofu, 1 tablespoon olive oil, 1/2 onion (chopped), 1 bell pepper (chopped), 1 cup spinach, 1/2 teaspoon turmeric, salt and pepper to taste.
 - Instructions:
1. Drain and crumble tofu.
2. Heat olive oil in a pan over medium heat.
3. Sauté onions and bell pepper until soft.
4. Add crumbled tofu, turmeric, salt, and pepper, and cook for 5-7 minutes.

5. Stir in spinach and cook until wilted.

6. Serve hot.

2. Southwest Tofu Scramble with Veggies

- Ingredients: 1 block firm tofu, 1 tablespoon olive oil, 1/2 onion (chopped), 1 jalapeño (chopped), 1 cup black beans, 1/2 teaspoon cumin, 1/2 teaspoon paprika, salt and pepper to taste.

- Instructions:

1. Drain and crumble tofu.

2. Heat olive oil in a pan over medium heat.

3. Sauté onions and jalapeño until soft.

4. Add crumbled tofu, cumin, paprika, salt, and pepper, and cook for 5-7 minutes.

5. Stir in black beans and heat through.

6. Serve hot.

3. Mediterranean Tofu Scramble with Veggies
   - Ingredients: 1 block firm tofu, 1 tablespoon olive oil, 1/2 onion (chopped), 1 zucchini (chopped), 1/2 cup cherry tomatoes (halved), 1/2 teaspoon oregano, salt and pepper to taste.
   - Instructions:
     1. Drain and crumble tofu.
     2. Heat olive oil in a pan over medium heat.
     3. Sauté onions and zucchini until soft.
     4. Add crumbled tofu, oregano, salt, and pepper, and cook for 5-7 minutes.
     5. Stir in cherry tomatoes and cook until soft.
     6. Serve hot.

4. Asian-Inspired Tofu Scramble with Veggies
   - Ingredients: 1 block firm tofu, 1 tablespoon sesame oil, 1/2 onion (chopped), 1 carrot (grated), 1 cup bok choy (chopped), 1 tablespoon soy sauce,

1/2 teaspoon ginger, salt and pepper to taste.

- Instructions:
1. Drain and crumble tofu.
2. Heat sesame oil in a pan over medium heat.
3. Sauté onions and carrot until soft.
4. Add crumbled tofu, soy sauce, ginger, salt, and pepper, and cook for 5-7 minutes.
5. Stir in bok choy and cook until wilted.
6. Serve hot.

Easy-to-Make Toasts

2. Spicy Avocado and Tomato Toast
- Ingredients: 1 ripe avocado, 2 slices whole-grain bread, 1 tomato (sliced), 1/2 teaspoon red pepper flakes, salt, pepper, lime juice.
- Instructions:
1. Toast the bread slices.

2. Mash the avocado in a bowl with lime juice, red pepper flakes, salt, and pepper.

3. Spread the avocado mixture on the toasted bread.

4. Top with tomato slices and sprinkle with extra red pepper flakes for added spice.

3. Herbed Avocado and Tomato Toast
   - Ingredients: 1 ripe avocado, 2 slices whole-grain bread, 1 tomato (sliced), 1 tablespoon fresh basil (chopped), salt, pepper, olive oil.
   - Instructions:
     1. Toast the bread slices.
     2. Mash the avocado in a bowl with a drizzle of olive oil, salt, and pepper.
     3. Spread the avocado mixture on the toasted bread.
     4. Top with tomato slices and sprinkle with chopped fresh basil.

4. Garlic Avocado and Tomato Toast

- Ingredients: 1 ripe avocado, 2 slices whole-grain bread, 1 tomato (sliced), 1 garlic clove (minced), salt, pepper, lemon juice.
- Instructions:
  1. Toast the bread slices.
  2. Mash the avocado in a bowl with lemon juice, minced garlic, salt, and pepper.
  3. Spread the avocado mixture on the toasted bread.
  4. Top with tomato slices and a pinch of salt and pepper.

Nut Butter and Apple Slices Toast
1. Classic Nut Butter and Apple Slices Toast
   - Ingredients: 2 slices whole-grain bread, 2 tablespoons almond butter, 1 apple (thinly sliced), cinnamon.
   - Instructions:
     1. Toast the bread slices.
     2. Spread almond butter evenly on each slice.
     3. Top with thin apple slices.

4. Sprinkle a dash of cinnamon over the apple slices.

2. Peanut Butter and Apple Slices Toast
   - Ingredients: 2 slices whole-grain bread, 2 tablespoons peanut butter, 1 apple (thinly sliced), honey.
   - Instructions:
   1. Toast the bread slices.
   2. Spread peanut butter evenly on each slice.
   3. Top with thin apple slices.
   4. Drizzle honey over the apple slices.

3. Cashew Butter and Apple Slices Toast
   - Ingredients: 2 slices whole-grain bread, 2 tablespoons cashew butter, 1 apple (thinly sliced), chia seeds.
   - Instructions:
   1. Toast the bread slices.
   2. Spread cashew butter evenly on each slice.
   3. Top with thin apple slices.
   4. Sprinkle chia seeds over the apple slices.

4. Sunflower Seed Butter and Apple Slices Toast

- Ingredients: 2 slices whole-grain bread, 2 tablespoons sunflower seed butter, 1 apple (thinly sliced), coconut flakes.
- Instructions:
1. Toast the bread slices.
2. Spread sunflower seed butter evenly on each slice.
3. Top with thin apple slices.
4. Sprinkle coconut flakes over the apple slices.

Lunch Recipes

Salads

Kidney-Friendly Kale Salad
1. Classic Kidney-Friendly Kale Salad
   - Ingredients:
     - 4 cups chopped kale
     - 1/2 cup shredded carrots

- 1/2 cup diced cucumber
- 1/4 cup chopped red bell pepper
- 1/4 cup sunflower seeds
- 1/4 cup dried cranberries (unsweetened)
- Dressing: 2 tablespoons olive oil, 1 tablespoon lemon juice, 1 teaspoon maple syrup, salt and pepper to taste.
- Instructions:

1. In a large bowl, combine the kale, carrots, cucumber, and red bell pepper.
2. In a small bowl, whisk together the olive oil, lemon juice, maple syrup, salt, and pepper.
3. Pour the dressing over the salad and toss well to coat.
4. Top with sunflower seeds and dried cranberries.
5. Serve immediately or chill for 15 minutes for the flavors to meld.

2. Berry Kale Salad
   - Ingredients:
     - 4 cups chopped kale
     - 1/2 cup sliced strawberries

- 1/4 cup blueberries
- 1/4 cup chopped walnuts
- 1/4 cup crumbled vegan feta cheese
- Dressing: 2 tablespoons balsamic vinegar, 1 tablespoon olive oil, 1 teaspoon agave syrup, salt and pepper to taste.
- Instructions:
1. In a large bowl, combine the kale, strawberries, blueberries, and walnuts.
2. In a small bowl, whisk together the balsamic vinegar, olive oil, agave syrup, salt, and pepper.
3. Pour the dressing over the salad and toss to coat.
4. Sprinkle with vegan feta cheese.
5. Serve immediately.

3. Apple and Pecan Kale Salad
 - Ingredients:
   - 4 cups chopped kale
   - 1 apple (thinly sliced)
   - 1/4 cup chopped pecans
   - 1/4 cup raisins

- Dressing: 2 tablespoons apple cider vinegar, 1 tablespoon olive oil, 1 teaspoon Dijon mustard, salt and pepper to taste.
- Instructions:
1. In a large bowl, combine the kale, apple slices, pecans, and raisins.
2. In a small bowl, whisk together the apple cider vinegar, olive oil, Dijon mustard, salt, and pepper.
3. Pour the dressing over the salad and toss to coat.
4. Serve immediately or let sit for 10 minutes to soften the kale.

4. Citrus Kale Salad
   - Ingredients:
     - 4 cups chopped kale
     - 1 orange (peeled and segmented)
     - 1/4 cup pomegranate seeds
     - 1/4 cup slivered almonds
     - Dressing: 2 tablespoons orange juice, 1 tablespoon olive oil, 1 teaspoon honey, salt and pepper to taste.
     - Instructions:

1. In a large bowl, combine the kale, orange segments, pomegranate seeds, and almonds.

2. In a small bowl, whisk together the orange juice, olive oil, honey, salt, and pepper.

3. Pour the dressing over the salad and toss to coat.

4. Serve immediately.

Quinoa and Black Bean Salad
1. Classic Quinoa and Black Bean Salad
   - Ingredients:
     - 1 cup cooked quinoa
     - 1 cup black beans (rinsed and drained)
     - 1/2 cup diced bell pepper
     - 1/2 cup diced tomato
     - 1/4 cup chopped cilantro
     - Dressing: 2 tablespoons lime juice, 1 tablespoon olive oil, 1 teaspoon cumin, salt and pepper to taste.
   - Instructions:

1. In a large bowl, combine the cooked quinoa, black beans, bell pepper, tomato, and cilantro.

2. In a small bowl, whisk together the lime juice, olive oil, cumin, salt, and pepper.

3. Pour the dressing over the salad and toss well to coat.

4. Serve immediately or chill for an hour for the flavors to meld.

2. Mango Quinoa and Black Bean Salad
   - Ingredients:
     - 1 cup cooked quinoa
     - 1 cup black beans (rinsed and drained)
     - 1 mango (diced)
     - 1/2 cup diced red onion
     - 1/4 cup chopped fresh mint
     - Dressing: 2 tablespoons lime juice, 1 tablespoon olive oil, 1 teaspoon agave syrup, salt and pepper to taste.
   - Instructions:

1. In a large bowl, combine the cooked quinoa, black beans, mango, red onion, and mint.

2. In a small bowl, whisk together the lime juice, olive oil, agave syrup, salt, and pepper.

3. Pour the dressing over the salad and toss to coat.

4. Serve immediately.

3. Southwest Quinoa and Black Bean Salad
  - Ingredients:
    - 1 cup cooked quinoa
    - 1 cup black beans (rinsed and drained)
    - 1/2 cup corn kernels (fresh or frozen, thawed)
    - 1/2 cup diced avocado
    - 1/4 cup chopped green onions
    - Dressing: 2 tablespoons lime juice, 1 tablespoon olive oil, 1 teaspoon chili powder, salt and pepper to taste.
  - Instructions:

1. In a large bowl, combine the cooked quinoa, black beans, corn, avocado, and green onions.
2. In a small bowl, whisk together the lime juice, olive oil, chili powder, salt, and pepper.
3. Pour the dressing over the salad and toss well to coat.
4. Serve immediately.

4. Mediterranean Quinoa and Black Bean Salad
   - Ingredients:
     - 1 cup cooked quinoa
     - 1 cup black beans (rinsed and drained)
     - 1/2 cup diced cucumber
     - 1/2 cup diced cherry tomatoes
     - 1/4 cup chopped fresh parsley
     - Dressing: 2 tablespoons lemon juice, 1 tablespoon olive oil, 1 teaspoon oregano, salt and pepper to taste.
   - Instructions:

1. In a large bowl, combine the cooked quinoa, black beans, cucumber, cherry tomatoes, and parsley.
2. In a small bowl, whisk together the lemon juice, olive oil, oregano, salt, and pepper.
3. Pour the dressing over the salad and toss to coat.
4. Serve immediately.

Soups

Lentil and Vegetable Soup
1. Classic Lentil and Vegetable Soup
   - Ingredients:
     - 1 cup dried lentils (rinsed)
     - 1 onion (chopped)
     - 2 carrots (diced)
     - 2 celery stalks (diced)
     - 1 zucchini (diced)
     - 4 cups vegetable broth
     - 2 cups water
     - 1 tablespoon olive oil
     - 1 teaspoon thyme
     - Salt and pepper to taste.

- Instructions:
  1. In a large pot, heat olive oil over medium heat.
  2. Add onion, carrots, and celery, and sauté until softened.
  3. Add lentils, vegetable broth, water, thyme, salt, and pepper.
  4. Bring to a boil, then reduce heat and simmer for 30 minutes.
  5. Add zucchini and cook for an additional 10 minutes until all vegetables are tender.
  6. Serve hot.

2. Spiced Lentil and Vegetable Soup
   - Ingredients:
     - 1 cup dried lentils (rinsed)
     - 1 onion (chopped)
     - 2 carrots (diced)
     - 2 celery stalks (diced)
     - 1 sweet potato (diced)
     - 4 cups vegetable broth
     - 2 cups water
     - 1 tablespoon olive oil
     - 1 teaspoon cumin

- 1 teaspoon turmeric
- Salt and pepper to taste.
- Instructions:
1. In a large pot, heat olive oil over medium heat.
2. Add onion, carrots, and celery, and sauté until softened.
3. Add lentils, vegetable broth, water, cumin, turmeric, salt, and pepper.
4. Bring to a boil, then reduce heat and simmer for 30 minutes.
5. Add sweet potato and cook for an additional 10 minutes until all vegetables are tender.
6. Serve hot.

3. Tomato Lentil and Vegetable Soup
   - Ingredients:
     - 1 cup dried lentils (rinsed)
     - 1 onion (chopped)
     - 2 carrots (diced)
     - 2 celery stalks (diced)
     - 1 can diced tomatoes (with juice)
     - 4 cups vegetable broth
     - 2 cups water

- 1 tablespoon olive oil
- 1 teaspoon basil
- Salt and pepper to taste.
- Instructions:
  1. In a large pot, heat olive oil over medium heat.
  2. Add onion, carrots, and celery, and sauté until softened.
  3. Add lentils, diced tomatoes with juice, vegetable broth, water, basil, salt, and pepper.
  4. Bring to a boil, then reduce heat and simmer for 30 minutes until lentils and vegetables are tender.
  5. Serve hot.

4. Hearty Lentil and Vegetable Soup
   - Ingredients:
     - 1 cup dried lentils (rinsed)
     - 1 onion (chopped)
     - 2 carrots (diced)
     - 2 celery stalks (diced)
     - 1 cup chopped kale
     - 4 cups vegetable broth
     - 2 cups water

- 1 tablespoon olive oil
- 1 teaspoon rosemary
- Salt and pepper to taste.
- Instructions:
1. In a large pot, heat olive oil over medium heat.
2. Add onion, carrots, and celery, and sauté until softened.
3. Add lentils, vegetable broth, water, rosemary, salt, and pepper.
4. Bring to a boil, then reduce heat and simmer for 30 minutes.
5. Add chopped kale and cook for an additional 10 minutes until kale is tender.
6. Serve hot.

Creamy Cauliflower Soup
1. Classic Creamy Cauliflower Soup
   - Ingredients:
     - 1 head of cauliflower (chopped)
     - 1 onion (chopped)
     - 2 garlic cloves (minced)
     - 4 cups vegetable broth
     - 1 cup unsweetened almond milk

- 2 tablespoons olive oil
- Salt and pepper to taste.
- Instructions:
1. In a large pot, heat olive oil over medium heat.
2. Add onion and garlic, and sauté until softened.
3. Add chopped cauliflower and vegetable broth.
4. Bring to a boil, then reduce heat and simmer for 20 minutes until cauliflower is tender.
5. Use an immersion blender to puree the soup until smooth.
6. Stir in almond milk, salt, and pepper.
7. Heat through and serve hot.

2. Roasted Garlic Cauliflower Soup
   - Ingredients:
     - 1 head of cauliflower (chopped)
     - 1 onion (chopped)
     - 1 bulb of garlic (roasted)
     - 4 cups vegetable broth
     - 1 cup unsweetened almond milk

- 2 tablespoons olive oil
- Salt and pepper to taste.
- Instructions:
  1. Preheat oven to 400°F (200°C).
  2. Cut the top off the garlic bulb, drizzle with olive oil, wrap in foil, and roast for 30-35 minutes until soft.
  3. In a large pot, heat olive oil over medium heat.
  4. Add onion and sauté until softened.
  5. Add chopped cauliflower and vegetable broth.
  6. Squeeze roasted garlic cloves into the pot.
  7. Bring to a boil, then reduce heat and simmer for 20 minutes until cauliflower is tender.
  8. Use an immersion blender to puree the soup until smooth.
  9. Stir in almond milk, salt, and pepper.
  10. Heat through and serve hot.

3. Spiced Cauliflower Soup

- Ingredients:
  - 1 head of cauliflower (chopped)
  - 1 onion (chopped)
  - 2 garlic cloves (minced)
  - 4 cups vegetable broth
  - 1 cup unsweetened coconut milk
  - 2 tablespoons olive oil
  - 1 teaspoon curry powder
  - 1/2 teaspoon turmeric
  - Salt and pepper to taste.
- Instructions:
  1. In a large pot, heat olive oil over medium heat.
  2. Add onion and garlic, and sauté until softened.
  3. Add curry powder and turmeric, and cook for 1 minute.
  4. Add chopped cauliflower and vegetable broth.
  5. Bring to a boil, then reduce heat and simmer for 20 minutes until cauliflower is tender.
  6. Use an immersion blender to puree the soup until smooth.

7. Stir in coconut milk, salt, and pepper.
8. Heat through and serve hot.

4. Cauliflower and Leek Soup
   - Ingredients:
     - 1 head of cauliflower (chopped)
     - 1 leek (sliced)
     - 2 garlic cloves (minced)
     - 4 cups vegetable broth
     - 1 cup unsweetened almond milk
     - 2 tablespoons olive oil
     - Salt and pepper to taste.
   - Instructions:
   1. In a large pot, heat olive oil over medium heat.
   2. Add sliced leek and garlic, and sauté until softened.
   3. Add chopped cauliflower and vegetable broth.
   4. Bring to a boil, then reduce heat and simmer for 20 minutes until cauliflower is tender.
   5. Use an immersion blender to puree the soup until smooth.

6. Stir in almond milk, salt, and pepper.

7. Heat through and serve hot.

Sandwiches and Wraps

Chickpea Salad Sandwich

1. Classic Chickpea Salad Sandwich
   - Ingredients:
     - 1 can chickpeas (rinsed and drained)
     - 1/4 cup vegan mayonnaise
     - 1 celery stalk (diced)
     - 1/4 cup diced red onion
     - 1 tablespoon lemon juice
     - Salt and pepper to taste
     - 4 slices whole-grain bread
     - Lettuce leaves.
   - Instructions:

1. In a bowl, mash the chickpeas with a fork until chunky.

2. Add vegan mayonnaise, celery, red onion, lemon juice, salt, and pepper. Mix well.

3. Spread the chickpea salad on two slices of bread.

4. Top with lettuce leaves and cover with the remaining bread slices.
5. Serve immediately.

2. Avocado Chickpea Salad Sandwich
   - Ingredients:
     - 1 can chickpeas (rinsed and drained)
     - 1 avocado (mashed)
     - 1/4 cup diced red bell pepper
     - 1 tablespoon lime juice
     - 1/4 teaspoon cumin
     - Salt and pepper to taste
     - 4 slices whole-grain bread
     - Spinach leaves.
   - Instructions:
     1. In a bowl, mash the chickpeas with a fork until chunky.
     2. Add mashed avocado, red bell pepper, lime juice, cumin, salt, and pepper. Mix well.
     3. Spread the chickpea salad on two slices of bread.
     4. Top with spinach leaves and cover with the remaining bread slices.
     5. Serve immediately.

3. Herbed Chickpea Salad Sandwich
   - Ingredients:
     - 1 can chickpeas (rinsed and drained)
     - 1/4 cup vegan mayonnaise
     - 1 tablespoon chopped fresh dill
     - 1 tablespoon chopped fresh parsley
     - 1 tablespoon lemon juice
     - Salt and pepper to taste
     - 4 slices whole-grain bread
     - Arugula leaves.
   - Instructions:
   1. In a bowl, mash the chickpeas with a fork until chunky.
   2. Add vegan mayonnaise, dill, parsley, lemon juice, salt, and pepper. Mix well.
   3. Spread the chickpea salad on two slices of bread.
   4. Top with arugula leaves and cover with the remaining bread slices.
   5. Serve immediately.

4. Spicy Chickpea Salad Sandwich
   - Ingredients:

- 1 can chickpeas (rinsed and drained)
- 1/4 cup vegan mayonnaise
- 1 tablespoon sriracha sauce
- 1/4 cup diced cucumber
- 1 tablespoon lime juice
- Salt and pepper to taste
- 4 slices whole-grain bread
- Romaine lettuce leaves.
- Instructions:

1. In a bowl, mash the chickpeas with a fork until chunky.
2. Add vegan mayonnaise, sriracha sauce, cucumber, lime juice, salt, and pepper. Mix well.
3. Spread the chickpea salad on two slices of bread.
4. Top with romaine lettuce leaves and cover with the remaining bread slices.
5. Serve immediately.

Hummus and Veggie Wrap
1. Classic Hummus and Veggie Wrap
    - Ingredients:
    - 1 large whole-grain tortilla

- 1/2 cup roasted red pepper hummus
- 1/4 cup chopped cherry tomatoes
- 1/4 cup sliced black olives
- 1/4 cup chopped cucumber
- Handful of spinach leaves.
- Instructions:
1. Spread roasted red pepper hummus evenly over the tortilla.
2. Layer chopped cherry tomatoes, black olives, cucumber, and spinach leaves on top.
3. Roll the tortilla tightly and slice in half.
4. Serve immediately or wrap in foil for later.

3. Spicy Hummus and Veggie Wrap
   - Ingredients:
     - 1 large whole-grain tortilla
     - 1/2 cup spicy hummus
     - 1/4 cup shredded lettuce
     - 1/4 cup julienned carrots
     - 1/4 cup sliced red bell pepper
     - 1/4 cup sliced avocado.
   - Instructions:

1. Spread spicy hummus evenly over the tortilla.
   2. Layer shredded lettuce, carrots, red bell pepper, and avocado slices on top.
   3. Roll the tortilla tightly and slice in half.
   4. Serve immediately or wrap in foil for later.

4. Creamy Hummus and Veggie Wrap
   - Ingredients:
     - 1 large whole-grain tortilla
     - 1/2 cup garlic hummus
     - 1/4 cup shredded cabbage
     - 1/4 cup grated beetroot
     - 1/4 cup sliced radishes
     - Handful of arugula.
   - Instructions:
   1. Spread garlic hummus evenly over the tortilla.
   2. Layer shredded cabbage, grated beetroot, sliced radishes, and arugula on top.
   3. Roll the tortilla tightly and slice in half.

4. Serve immediately or wrap in foil for later.

These lunch recipes not only provide variety but also ensure that your meals are packed with kidney-friendly nutrients while being delicious and satisfying. Whether you prefer a refreshing salad, a warm soup, or a hearty sandwich or wrap, there's something here to delight your taste buds and support your kidney health.

Dinner Recipes

Hearty Main Dishes

Stuffed Bell Peppers
1. Classic Stuffed Bell Peppers
   - Ingredients:
     - 4 large bell peppers (tops cut off, seeds removed)
     - 1 cup cooked quinoa
     - 1 can black beans (rinsed and drained)
     - 1 cup corn kernels
     - 1/2 cup diced tomatoes
     - 1/4 cup chopped cilantro
     - 1 tablespoon olive oil
     - 1 teaspoon cumin
     - Salt and pepper to taste.
   - Instructions:
     1. Preheat oven to 375°F (190°C).
     2. In a bowl, mix quinoa, black beans, corn, diced tomatoes, cilantro, olive oil, cumin, salt, and pepper.
     3. Stuff each bell pepper with the quinoa mixture.

4. Place the stuffed peppers in a baking dish and cover with foil.
5. Bake for 35-40 minutes until peppers are tender.
6. Serve hot.

2. Mexican-Inspired Stuffed Bell Peppers
   - Ingredients:
     - 4 large bell peppers (tops cut off, seeds removed)
     - 1 cup cooked brown rice
     - 1 can pinto beans (rinsed and drained)
     - 1 cup salsa
     - 1/2 cup corn kernels
     - 1 teaspoon chili powder
     - 1 teaspoon paprika
     - Salt and pepper to taste.
   - Instructions:
     1. Preheat oven to 375°F (190°C).
     2. In a bowl, mix brown rice, pinto beans, salsa, corn, chili powder, paprika, salt, and pepper.

3. Stuff each bell pepper with the rice mixture.

4. Place the stuffed peppers in a baking dish and cover with foil.

5. Bake for 35-40 minutes until peppers are tender.

6. Serve hot.

3. Mediterranean Stuffed Bell Peppers
 - Ingredients:
   - 4 large bell peppers (tops cut off, seeds removed)
   - 1 cup cooked couscous
   - 1/2 cup diced cucumber
   - 1/2 cup cherry tomatoes (halved)
   - 1/4 cup chopped Kalamata olives
   - 1/4 cup chopped parsley
   - 2 tablespoons lemon juice
   - 2 tablespoons olive oil
   - Salt and pepper to taste.
 - Instructions:
   1. Preheat oven to 375°F (190°C).
   2. In a bowl, mix couscous, cucumber, cherry tomatoes, olives, parsley, lemon juice, olive oil, salt, and pepper.

3. Stuff each bell pepper with the couscous mixture.
4. Place the stuffed peppers in a baking dish and cover with foil.
5. Bake for 35-40 minutes until peppers are tender.
6. Serve hot.

4. Italian Stuffed Bell Peppers
   - Ingredients:
     - 4 large bell peppers (tops cut off, seeds removed)
     - 1 cup cooked farro
     - 1 cup marinara sauce
     - 1/2 cup diced zucchini
     - 1/2 cup diced mushrooms
     - 1 teaspoon dried oregano
     - 1 teaspoon dried basil
     - Salt and pepper to taste.
   - Instructions:
     1. Preheat oven to 375°F (190°C).
     2. In a bowl, mix farro, marinara sauce, zucchini, mushrooms, oregano, basil, salt, and pepper.

3. Stuff each bell pepper with the farro mixture.

4. Place the stuffed peppers in a baking dish and cover with foil.

5. Bake for 35-40 minutes until peppers are tender.

6. Serve hot.

Baked Eggplant Parmesan
1. Classic Baked Eggplant Parmesan
   - Ingredients:
     - 1 large eggplant (sliced into 1/2-inch rounds)
     - 1 cup breadcrumbs
     - 1/2 cup nutritional yeast
     - 1 cup marinara sauce
     - 1 cup shredded vegan mozzarella
     - 1/4 cup chopped fresh basil
     - 2 tablespoons olive oil
     - Salt and pepper to taste.
   - Instructions:
     1. Preheat oven to 375°F (190°C).
     2. Brush eggplant slices with olive oil and season with salt and pepper.

3. Mix breadcrumbs and nutritional yeast in a bowl.
4. Dredge each eggplant slice in the breadcrumb mixture, coating evenly.
5. Place the coated slices on a baking sheet and bake for 20 minutes, flipping halfway through.
6. Spread a thin layer of marinara sauce in a baking dish.
7. Layer the eggplant slices, marinara sauce, and vegan mozzarella.
8. Repeat layers, ending with a layer of vegan mozzarella.
9. Bake for 25-30 minutes until bubbly and golden.
10. Garnish with fresh basil and serve hot.

2. Spinach and Mushroom Baked Eggplant Parmesan
   - Ingredients:
   - 1 large eggplant (sliced into 1/2-inch rounds)
   - 1 cup breadcrumbs
   - 1/2 cup nutritional yeast

- 1 cup marinara sauce
- 1 cup shredded vegan mozzarella
- 1/2 cup sautéed spinach
- 1/2 cup sautéed mushrooms
- 2 tablespoons olive oil
- Salt and pepper to taste.
- Instructions:
1. Preheat oven to 375°F (190°C).
2. Brush eggplant slices with olive oil and season with salt and pepper.
3. Mix breadcrumbs and nutritional yeast in a bowl.
4. Dredge each eggplant slice in the breadcrumb mixture, coating evenly.
5. Place the coated slices on a baking sheet and bake for 20 minutes, flipping halfway through.
6. Spread a thin layer of marinara sauce in a baking dish.
7. Layer the eggplant slices, sautéed spinach, sautéed mushrooms, marinara sauce, and vegan mozzarella.
8. Repeat layers, ending with a layer of vegan mozzarella.

9. Bake for 25-30 minutes until bubbly and golden.

10. Serve hot.

3. Pesto Baked Eggplant Parmesan
   - Ingredients:
     - 1 large eggplant (sliced into 1/2-inch rounds)
     - 1 cup breadcrumbs
     - 1/2 cup nutritional yeast
     - 1 cup marinara sauce
     - 1 cup shredded vegan mozzarella
     - 1/2 cup vegan pesto
     - 2 tablespoons olive oil
     - Salt and pepper to taste.
   - Instructions:
     1. Preheat oven to 375°F (190°C).
     2. Brush eggplant slices with olive oil and season with salt and pepper.
     3. Mix breadcrumbs and nutritional yeast in a bowl.
     4. Dredge each eggplant slice in the breadcrumb mixture, coating evenly.

5. Place the coated slices on a baking sheet and bake for 20 minutes, flipping halfway through.

6. Spread a thin layer of marinara sauce in a baking dish.

7. Layer the eggplant slices, vegan pesto, marinara sauce, and vegan mozzarella.

8. Repeat layers, ending with a layer of vegan mozzarella.

9. Bake for 25-30 minutes until bubbly and golden.

10. Serve hot.

4. Roasted Red Pepper Baked Eggplant Parmesan
  - Ingredients:
    - 1 large eggplant (sliced into 1/2-inch rounds)
    - 1 cup breadcrumbs
    - 1/2 cup nutritional yeast
    - 1 cup marinara sauce
    - 1 cup shredded vegan mozzarella
    - 1/2 cup roasted red peppers (sliced)
    - 2 tablespoons olive oil

- Salt and pepper to taste.
- Instructions:
1. Preheat oven to 375°F (190°C).
2. Brush eggplant slices with olive oil and season with salt and pepper.
3. Mix breadcrumbs and nutritional yeast in a bowl.
4. Dredge each eggplant slice in the breadcrumb mixture, coating evenly.
5. Place the coated slices on a baking sheet and bake for 20 minutes, flipping halfway through.
6. Spread a thin layer of marinara sauce in a baking dish.
7. Layer the eggplant slices, roasted red peppers, marinara sauce, and vegan mozzarella.
8. Repeat layers, ending with a layer of vegan mozzarella.
9. Bake for 25-30 minutes until bubbly and golden.
10. Serve hot.

Pasta and Noodles

Zucchini Noodles with Pesto

1. Classic Zucchini Noodles with Pesto
   - Ingredients:
     - 4 medium zucchinis (spiralized)
     - 1 cup fresh basil leaves
     - 1/4 cup pine nuts
     - 2 garlic cloves
     - 1/4 cup nutritional yeast
     - 1/4 cup olive oil
     - Salt and pepper to taste.
   - Instructions:
     1. Spiralize the zucchinis and set aside.
     2. In a food processor, combine basil leaves, pine nuts, garlic cloves, nutritional yeast, olive oil, salt, and pepper. Blend until smooth to make the pesto.
     3. Toss the zucchini noodles with the pesto until evenly coated.
     4. Serve immediately or chill for a cold dish.

2. Zucchini Noodles with Avocado Pesto
   - Ingredients:

- 4 medium zucchinis (spiralized)
- 2 ripe avocados
- 1 cup fresh basil leaves
- 1/4 cup pine nuts
- 2 garlic cloves
- Juice of 1 lemon
- 1/4 cup olive oil
- Salt and pepper to taste.
- Instructions:
1. Spiralize the zucchinis and set aside.
2. In a food processor, combine avocados, basil leaves, pine nuts, garlic cloves, lemon juice, olive oil, salt, and pepper. Blend until smooth to make the avocado pesto.
3. Toss the zucchini noodles with the avocado pesto until evenly coated.
4. Serve immediately or chill for a cold dish.

3. Zucchini Noodles with Sun-Dried Tomato Pesto
   - Ingredients:
     - 4 medium zucchinis (spiralized)

- 1 cup sun-dried tomatoes (packed in oil)
- 1/4 cup fresh basil leaves
- 2 garlic cloves
- 1/4 cup nutritional yeast
- 1/4 cup olive oil
- Salt and pepper to taste.
- Instructions:

1. Spiralize the zucchinis and set aside.
2. In a food processor, combine sun-dried tomatoes, basil leaves, garlic cloves, nutritional yeast, olive oil, salt, and pepper. Blend until smooth to make the sun-dried tomato pesto.
3. Toss the zucchini noodles with the sun-dried tomato pesto until evenly coated.
4. Serve immediately or chill for a cold dish.

4. Zucchini Noodles with Spinach Pesto
   - Ingredients:
     - 4 medium zucchinis (spiralized)
     - 1 cup fresh spinach leaves

- 1/4 cup walnuts
- 2 garlic cloves
- 1/4 cup nutritional yeast
- 1/4 cup olive oil
- Salt and pepper to taste.
- Instructions:
1. Spiralize the zucchinis and set aside.
2. In a food processor, combine spinach leaves, walnuts, garlic cloves, nutritional yeast, olive oil, salt, and pepper. Blend until smooth to make the spinach pesto.
3. Toss the zucchini noodles with the spinach pesto until evenly coated.
4. Serve immediately or chill for a cold dish.

Vegan Mac and Cheese
1. Classic Vegan Mac and Cheese
   - Ingredients:
     - 8 ounces elbow macaroni
     - 1 cup raw cashews (soaked for at least 4 hours)
     - 1 cup unsweetened almond milk

- 1/4 cup nutritional yeast
- 1 teaspoon garlic powder
- 1 teaspoon onion powder
- 1 tablespoon lemon juice
- Salt and pepper to taste.
- Instructions:
  1. Cook the elbow macaroni according to package instructions.
  2. In a blender, combine soaked cashews, almond milk, nutritional yeast, garlic powder, onion powder, lemon juice, salt, and pepper. Blend until smooth to make the cheese sauce.
  3. Drain the macaroni and return it to the pot.
  4. Pour the cheese sauce over the macaroni and stir to combine.
  5. Heat on low until warmed through.
  6. Serve hot.

2. Butternut Squash Vegan Mac and Cheese
   - Ingredients:
     - 8 ounces elbow macaroni

- 1 cup cooked butternut squash (mashed)
- 1 cup unsweetened almond milk
- 1/4 cup nutritional yeast
- 1 teaspoon garlic powder
- 1 teaspoon onion powder
- 1 tablespoon lemon juice
- Salt and pepper to taste.
- Instructions:

1. Cook the elbow macaroni according to package instructions.
2. In a blender, combine mashed butternut squash, almond milk, nutritional yeast, garlic powder, onion powder, lemon juice, salt, and pepper. Blend until smooth to make the cheese sauce.
3. Drain the macaroni and return it to the pot.
4. Pour the cheese sauce over the macaroni and stir to combine.
5. Heat on low until warmed through.
6. Serve hot.

3. Pumpkin Vegan Mac and Cheese

- Ingredients:
  - 8 ounces elbow macaroni
  - 1 cup pumpkin puree
  - 1 cup unsweetened almond milk
  - 1/4 cup nutritional yeast
  - 1 teaspoon garlic powder
  - 1 teaspoon onion powder
  - 1 tablespoon lemon juice
  - Salt and pepper to taste.
- Instructions:
  1. Cook the elbow macaroni according to package instructions.
  2. In a blender, combine pumpkin puree, almond milk, nutritional yeast, garlic powder, onion powder, lemon juice, salt, and pepper. Blend until smooth to make the cheese sauce.
  3. Drain the macaroni and return it to the pot.
  4. Pour the cheese sauce over the macaroni and stir to combine.
  5. Heat on low until warmed through.
  6. Serve hot.

4. Cauliflower Vegan Mac and Cheese

- Ingredients:
  - 8 ounces elbow macaroni
  - 1 cup steamed cauliflower florets
  - 1 cup unsweetened almond milk
  - 1/4 cup nutritional yeast
  - 1 teaspoon garlic powder
  - 1 teaspoon onion powder
  - 1 tablespoon lemon juice
  - Salt and pepper to taste.
- Instructions:
  1. Cook the elbow macaroni according to package instructions.
  2. In a blender, combine steamed cauliflower, almond milk, nutritional yeast, garlic powder, onion powder, lemon juice, salt, and pepper. Blend until smooth to make the cheese sauce.
  3. Drain the macaroni and return it to the pot.
  4. Pour the cheese sauce over the macaroni and stir to combine.
  5. Heat on low until warmed through.
  6. Serve hot.

Casseroles and Bakes

Sweet Potato and Black Bean Casserole
1. Classic Sweet Potato and Black Bean Casserole
  - Ingredients:
    - 2 large sweet potatoes (peeled and diced)
    - 1 can black beans (rinsed and drained)
    - 1 cup corn kernels
    - 1 cup salsa
    - 1 teaspoon cumin
    - 1 teaspoon chili powder
    - 1/2 cup shredded vegan cheese
    - Salt and pepper to taste.
  - Instructions:
    1. Preheat oven to 375°F (190°C).
    2. In a large bowl, combine sweet potatoes, black beans, corn, salsa, cumin, chili powder, salt, and pepper.
    3. Transfer the mixture to a baking dish and spread evenly.
    4. Top with shredded vegan cheese.
    5. Cover with foil and bake for 30-35 minutes, until sweet potatoes are tender.

6. Remove the foil and bake for an additional 10 minutes, until the cheese is melted and bubbly.

7. Serve hot.

2. Mexican Sweet Potato and Black Bean Casserole
- Ingredients:
- 2 large sweet potatoes (peeled and diced)
- 1 can black beans (rinsed and drained)
- 1 cup corn kernels
- 1 cup salsa
- 1/2 cup chopped bell pepper
- 1 teaspoon cumin
- 1 teaspoon smoked paprika
- 1/2 cup shredded vegan cheese
- Salt and pepper to taste.
- Instructions:

1. Preheat oven to 375°F (190°C).

2. In a large bowl, combine sweet potatoes, black beans, corn, salsa, bell pepper, cumin, smoked paprika, salt, and pepper.

3. Transfer the mixture to a baking dish and spread evenly.

4. Top with shredded vegan cheese.

5. Cover with foil and bake for 30-35 minutes, until sweet potatoes are tender.

6. Remove the foil and bake for an additional 10 minutes, until the cheese is melted and bubbly.

7. Serve hot.

Desserts

Kidney-Friendly Sweet Treats

Chia Seed Pudding
1. Classic Chia Seed Pudding
   - Ingredients:
     - 1/4 cup chia seeds
     - 1 cup unsweetened almond milk
     - 1 tablespoon maple syrup
     - 1/2 teaspoon vanilla extract
   - Instructions:
     1. In a bowl, combine chia seeds, almond milk, maple syrup, and vanilla extract.
     2. Stir well to ensure the chia seeds are evenly distributed.
     3. Cover and refrigerate for at least 4 hours or overnight.
     4. Stir again before serving and top with fresh fruit or nuts if desired.

2. Berry Chia Seed Pudding
   - Ingredients:
     - 1/4 cup chia seeds
     - 1 cup unsweetened almond milk
     - 1 tablespoon maple syrup
     - 1/2 teaspoon vanilla extract
     - 1/2 cup mixed berries (fresh or frozen)
   - Instructions:
     1. In a bowl, combine chia seeds, almond milk, maple syrup, and vanilla extract.
     2. Stir well to ensure the chia seeds are evenly distributed.
     3. Add the mixed berries and stir again.
     4. Cover and refrigerate for at least 4 hours or overnight.
     5. Stir before serving and enjoy.

Apple and Cinnamon Bites
1. Classic Apple and Cinnamon Bites
   - Ingredients:
     - 2 apples (cored and sliced)
     - 1 tablespoon lemon juice

- 1 teaspoon ground cinnamon
- 1 tablespoon maple syrup
- Instructions:
  1. Preheat oven to 350°F (175°C).
  2. Toss apple slices with lemon juice to prevent browning.
  3. Arrange the apple slices on a baking sheet lined with parchment paper.
  4. Sprinkle ground cinnamon and drizzle maple syrup over the apple slices.
  5. Bake for 15-20 minutes until the apples are tender.
  6. Let cool slightly before serving.

2. Apple and Cinnamon Energy Bites
   - Ingredients:
     - 1 cup dried apples (chopped)
     - 1/2 cup oats
     - 1/4 cup almond butter
     - 1 tablespoon maple syrup
     - 1 teaspoon ground cinnamon
     - 1/4 cup shredded coconut (optional)
   - Instructions:

1. In a food processor, combine dried apples, oats, almond butter, maple syrup, and ground cinnamon.
2. Pulse until the mixture comes together and forms a sticky dough.
3. Roll the mixture into small bite-sized balls.
4. Optional: Roll the bites in shredded coconut.
5. Place the energy bites on a baking sheet and refrigerate for at least 30 minutes before serving.

Baking Delights

Banana Oatmeal Cookies
1. Classic Banana Oatmeal Cookies
   - Ingredients:
     - 2 ripe bananas (mashed)
     - 1 1/2 cups rolled oats
     - 1/2 cup almond butter
     - 1/4 cup maple syrup
     - 1/2 teaspoon vanilla extract
     - 1/2 teaspoon ground cinnamon

- 1/4 cup dark chocolate chips (optional)
- Instructions:
1. Preheat oven to 350°F (175°C).
2. In a large bowl, combine mashed bananas, rolled oats, almond butter, maple syrup, vanilla extract, and ground cinnamon. Mix well.
3. Optional: Fold in dark chocolate chips.
4. Drop spoonfuls of dough onto a baking sheet lined with parchment paper.
5. Flatten each cookie slightly with the back of a spoon.
6. Bake for 12-15 minutes until golden brown.
7. Let cool on a wire rack before serving.

2. Banana Oatmeal Raisin Cookies
   - Ingredients:
     - 2 ripe bananas (mashed)
     - 1 1/2 cups rolled oats
     - 1/2 cup almond butter

- 1/4 cup maple syrup
- 1/2 teaspoon vanilla extract
- 1/2 teaspoon ground cinnamon
- 1/4 cup raisins
- Instructions:
1. Preheat oven to 350°F (175°C).
2. In a large bowl, combine mashed bananas, rolled oats, almond butter, maple syrup, vanilla extract, and ground cinnamon. Mix well.
3. Fold in raisins.
4. Drop spoonfuls of dough onto a baking sheet lined with parchment paper.
5. Flatten each cookie slightly with the back of a spoon.
6. Bake for 12-15 minutes until golden brown.
7. Let cool on a wire rack before serving.

Vegan Brownies
1. Classic Vegan Brownies
   - Ingredients:
     - 1 cup all-purpose flour

- 1 cup granulated sugar
- 1/2 cup cocoa powder
- 1 teaspoon baking powder
- 1/2 teaspoon salt
- 1/2 cup unsweetened almond milk
- 1/2 cup vegetable oil
- 1 teaspoon vanilla extract
- 1/2 cup dark chocolate chips (optional)
- Instructions:
1. Preheat oven to 350°F (175°C).
2. In a large bowl, whisk together flour, sugar, cocoa powder, baking powder, and salt.
3. Add almond milk, vegetable oil, and vanilla extract to the dry ingredients. Mix until well combined.
4. Optional: Fold in dark chocolate chips.
5. Pour the batter into a greased 8x8-inch baking dish.
6. Bake for 20-25 minutes until a toothpick inserted in the center comes out clean.

7. Let cool before cutting into squares and serving.

2. Avocado Vegan Brownies
   - Ingredients:
     - 1 cup all-purpose flour
     - 1 cup granulated sugar
     - 1/2 cup cocoa powder
     - 1 teaspoon baking powder
     - 1/2 teaspoon salt
     - 1 ripe avocado (mashed)
     - 1/2 cup unsweetened almond milk
     - 1/4 cup vegetable oil
     - 1 teaspoon vanilla extract
     - 1/2 cup dark chocolate chips (optional)
   - Instructions:
     1. Preheat oven to 350°F (175°C).
     2. In a large bowl, whisk together flour, sugar, cocoa powder, baking powder, and salt.
     3. Add mashed avocado, almond milk, vegetable oil, and vanilla extract to the dry ingredients. Mix until well combined.

4. Optional: Fold in dark chocolate chips.

5. Pour the batter into a greased 8x8-inch baking dish.

6. Bake for 20-25 minutes until a toothpick inserted in the center comes out clean.

7. Let cool before cutting into squares and serving.

Hydration Tips for Kidney Health

Staying hydrated is essential for kidney health. The kidneys play a crucial role in filtering waste products from the blood and maintaining overall fluid balance in the body. Proper hydration helps to ensure that your kidneys can perform these functions effectively. Here, we'll explore some delicious and kidney-friendly hydration options, including smoothies, juices, and herbal teas. We'll also discuss practical tips for incorporating these beverages into your daily routine, considering the busy lives we lead.

Smoothies and Juices

Green Detox Juice

A refreshing and nutrient-packed green detox juice can be a fantastic way to start your day. Not only does it hydrate you, but it also provides essential vitamins and minerals that support kidney function.

- Ingredients:
  - 1 cucumber
  - 2 celery stalks
  - 1 green apple
  - 1/2 lemon (juiced)
  - A handful of spinach
  - A small piece of ginger
  - 1 cup water

- Instructions:
  1. Wash all the ingredients thoroughly.
  2. Cut the cucumber, celery, and apple into smaller pieces.
  3. Add all the ingredients to a blender, along with the water.
  4. Blend until smooth.
  5. Strain the juice through a fine mesh sieve or cheesecloth if you prefer a smoother texture.

6. Serve immediately and enjoy the refreshing taste.

Practical Tips:
- Morning Boost: Prepare this juice in the morning to kickstart your day. It's quick to make and can be consumed while you're getting ready for work or other activities.
- Batch Preparation: If mornings are particularly hectic, prepare a larger batch the night before. Store it in the refrigerator in an airtight container and give it a good shake before drinking.

Berry Blast Smoothie

Smoothies are not only hydrating but also a great way to pack in nutrients. This berry blast smoothie is rich in antioxidants, which are beneficial for overall health, including kidney function.

- Ingredients:

- 1 cup mixed berries (strawberries, blueberries, raspberries)
- 1/2 banana
- 1 cup unsweetened almond milk
- 1 tablespoon chia seeds
- 1/2 teaspoon vanilla extract (optional)

- Instructions:
1. Combine all the ingredients in a blender.
2. Blend until smooth and creamy.
3. Pour into a glass and enjoy immediately.

Practical Tips:
- On-the-Go: This smoothie can be a quick breakfast or snack option. Pour it into a travel-friendly container, and you have a nutritious drink to enjoy on your commute or at your desk.
- Frozen Berries: Using frozen berries can make the smoothie colder and more refreshing. Plus, they're available year-round and often more economical.

Herbal Teas and Infusions

Lemon Ginger Tea

Lemon ginger tea is not only hydrating but also soothing. Ginger has anti-inflammatory properties, and lemon provides a good dose of vitamin C, which is beneficial for overall health.

- Ingredients:
  - 1 inch piece of fresh ginger (sliced)
  - 1/2 lemon (sliced)
  - 2 cups water
  - Honey (optional, for taste)

- Instructions:
  1. Boil the water in a saucepan.
  2. Add the ginger slices and let it simmer for about 10 minutes.
  3. Remove from heat and add the lemon slices.
  4. Let it steep for a few minutes.
  5. Strain into a cup and add honey if desired.

6. Enjoy warm or let it cool and serve over ice for a refreshing iced tea.

Practical Tips:
- Evening Relaxation: This tea is perfect for winding down in the evening. Its soothing properties can help you relax after a long day.
- Thermos Trick: Make a larger batch and keep it in a thermos. This way, you can have it warm throughout the day without needing to reheat.

Hibiscus Iced Tea

Hibiscus tea is not only hydrating but also known for its ability to help maintain healthy blood pressure levels. It's a beautiful, deep red tea that's naturally tart and refreshing.

- Ingredients:
    - 2 tablespoons dried hibiscus flowers
    - 4 cups water
    - Sweetener of choice (optional)

- Instructions:
  1. Bring the water to a boil.
  2. Remove from heat and add the dried hibiscus flowers.
  3. Let it steep for about 10 minutes.
  4. Strain the tea into a pitcher and let it cool.
  5. Add sweetener if desired.
  6. Serve over ice for a refreshing drink.

Practical Tips:
- Hydration with a Twist: This iced tea can be a delightful alternative to plain water. Keep a pitcher in your refrigerator, and you'll have a refreshing drink ready whenever you need it.
- Flavor Variations: Experiment by adding slices of orange, mint leaves, or a splash of sparkling water to change up the flavor.

Practical Hydration Tips

Start Your Day Hydrated

- Morning Routine: Begin your day with a glass of water. This simple habit can help kickstart your metabolism and get your kidneys functioning optimally after a night's rest.
- Infused Water: If plain water isn't appealing, infuse it with slices of cucumber, lemon, or berries for added flavor and nutrients.

Carry a Water Bottle
- Always Accessible: Carrying a reusable water bottle ensures you have water available wherever you go. This can help you stay hydrated throughout the day without needing to purchase bottled drinks.
- Track Your Intake: Many modern water bottles come with measurements or time markers to help you track how much water you're drinking.

Hydration Reminders
- Set Alarms: Use your phone to set hourly reminders to take a sip of water.

This can be especially helpful if you have a busy schedule.
- Hydration Apps: There are several apps available that can help track your water intake and remind you to drink throughout the day.

Eat Hydrating Foods
- Fruits and Vegetables: Incorporate high-water-content foods into your diet, such as cucumbers, watermelon, oranges, and strawberries. These foods not only provide hydration but also essential vitamins and minerals.
- Soups and Broths: Including a kidney-friendly soup or broth in your daily meals can boost your overall fluid intake.

Adjust for Activity Levels
- Increased Hydration Needs: If you exercise regularly or live in a hot climate, your hydration needs will be higher. Ensure you drink extra water to

compensate for the fluids lost through sweat.

- Post-Exercise: After a workout, replenish your fluids with water or a hydrating smoothie. Avoid sugary sports drinks that can add unnecessary calories and chemicals.

Conclusion

Maintaining proper hydration is vital for kidney health and overall well-being. By incorporating hydrating beverages like green detox juices, berry smoothies, and herbal teas into your daily routine, you can ensure that your kidneys function efficiently. These drinks are not only beneficial for hydration but also packed with nutrients that support kidney health. Remember to start your day with water, carry a reusable bottle, set hydration reminders, eat hydrating foods, and adjust your intake based on your activity levels. With these practical tips, you can easily stay hydrated and support your kidney health throughout the day.

Meal Planning and Preparation

Alright, let's dive into the art of meal planning and preparation. Trust me, mastering this will not only make your life easier but also ensure you're eating healthy, kidney-friendly meals without the daily hassle of figuring out what's for dinner. We'll go through weekly meal plans, batch cooking tips, and the best ways to store and reheat your meals. Grab a cup of tea, and let's get started!

Weekly Meal Plans

Creating a weekly meal plan is like setting up a roadmap for your week's eating. It takes a bit of upfront effort but saves you tons of time and stress during the week. Here's how to craft a plan that works for you:

1. Start with a Template: Find or create a simple weekly meal planning template. It can be digital or a printed version that you stick on your fridge. Divide it into days of the week and include slots for breakfast, lunch, dinner, and snacks.

2. Choose Your Recipes: Spend some time selecting recipes that you enjoy and that align with your dietary needs. For a kidney-friendly, vegan diet, you might want to include a mix of smoothies, salads, soups, hearty main dishes, and a few delightful snacks. Balance is key.

3. Check Your Pantry: Before you finalize your plan, check what ingredients you already have. This helps you avoid buying duplicates and keeps your kitchen clutter-free. Make a shopping list for the items you need to buy.

4. Plan for Leftovers: Be smart about your choices. Plan to cook larger

portions of certain meals that can be eaten as leftovers. This saves cooking time and ensures you have ready-to-eat meals for those busy days.

5. Variety is Vital: Mix up your meals to avoid monotony. If you had a smoothie for breakfast on Monday, maybe go for oatmeal or a breakfast bowl on Tuesday. This keeps things exciting and ensures a broader range of nutrients.

Here's a sample weekly meal plan to get you started:

- Monday
  - Breakfast: Berry-Spinach Smoothie
  - Lunch: Quinoa and Black Bean Salad
  - Dinner: Baked Eggplant Parmesan
  - Snack: Apple and Cinnamon Bites

- Tuesday
  - Breakfast: Almond Butter Banana Shake
  - Lunch: Creamy Cauliflower Soup

- Dinner: Sweet Potato and Black Bean Casserole
- Snack: Banana Oatmeal Cookies

- Wednesday
  - Breakfast: Quinoa Porridge with Berries
  - Lunch: Lentil and Vegetable Soup
  - Dinner: Zucchini Noodles with Pesto
  - Snack: Chia Seed Pudding

- Thursday
  - Breakfast: Tofu Scramble with Veggies
  - Lunch: Kidney-Friendly Kale Salad
  - Dinner: Stuffed Bell Peppers
  - Snack: Vegan Brownies

- Friday
  - Breakfast: Avocado and Tomato Toast
  - Lunch: Chickpea Salad Sandwich
  - Dinner: Vegan Mac and Cheese
  - Snack: Berry Blast Smoothie

- Saturday

- Breakfast: Nut Butter and Apple Slices Toast
- Lunch: Hummus and Veggie Wrap
- Dinner: Vegetable Lasagna
- Snack: Lemon Ginger Tea

- Sunday
  - Breakfast: Green Detox Juice
  - Lunch: Lentil and Vegetable Soup (leftovers)
  - Dinner: Sweet Potato and Black Bean Casserole (leftovers)
  - Snack: Hibiscus Iced Tea

Tips for Batch Cooking

Batch cooking is a lifesaver, especially when you have a busy schedule. It allows you to prepare large quantities of food in one go, so you have ready-to-eat meals throughout the week. Here's how to do it effectively:

1. Plan Your Batch Cooking Day: Choose a day when you have a few hours to

spare. Many people prefer Sundays, but any day that fits your schedule works.

2. Prep Ingredients First: Before you start cooking, prep all your ingredients. Chop veggies, cook grains, and measure out spices. This makes the actual cooking process smoother and faster.

3. Use Your Oven and Stovetop Efficiently: Cook multiple dishes at the same time. For example, while your Sweet Potato and Black Bean Casserole is baking in the oven, you can simmer Lentil and Vegetable Soup on the stovetop. Multi-tasking is your friend here.

4. Double Up: If you're already making a dish, why not double the recipe? This way, you can freeze half for future use. It's the same effort with twice the reward.

5. Invest in Good Containers: Store your meals in high-quality, airtight containers. Glass containers are great because they're microwave safe and don't retain odors. Label them with the date and contents to keep track of what needs to be eaten first.

6. Stay Organized: Keep a list of the meals you've prepped and stored in the fridge or freezer. This helps you remember what you have and plan your meals accordingly.

7. Clean as You Go: To avoid a huge cleanup job at the end, clean up as you cook. Wash utensils and bowls as you finish using them. This keeps your workspace tidy and makes the whole process more enjoyable.

Storing and Reheating

Storing and reheating your meals properly ensures they stay fresh and safe to eat. Here's how to do it right:

1. Cool Before Storing: Let hot foods cool to room temperature before storing them in the fridge or freezer. This prevents condensation and helps your fridge maintain a stable temperature.

2. Use the Right Containers: As mentioned earlier, airtight containers are essential. For freezing, consider using containers that are specifically designed for freezer storage, as they help prevent freezer burn.

3. Portion Control: Store your meals in single-serving portions. This makes it easier to reheat just the amount you need and helps with portion control.

4. Label Everything: Always label your containers with the date and contents. Use a piece of masking tape and a

permanent marker for easy labeling. This helps you keep track of how long something has been stored.

5. Reheat Safely: When reheating, ensure that the food is heated thoroughly. The internal temperature should reach at least 165°F (74°C) to kill any potential bacteria. Stir soups and casseroles halfway through heating to ensure even distribution of heat.

6. Microwave Tips: Cover your food with a microwave-safe lid or a damp paper towel to prevent splatters and retain moisture. If reheating from frozen, use the defrost setting first before fully reheating.

7. Oven Reheating: For dishes like casseroles and baked goods, reheating in the oven can help maintain their texture. Preheat the oven to 350°F (175°C) and cover the dish with foil to prevent it

from drying out. Reheat until the dish is hot all the way through.

8. Stovetop Reheating: Soups and stews reheat well on the stovetop. Heat them over medium heat, stirring occasionally, until they're hot throughout. Adding a bit of water or broth can help if the soup has thickened too much.

Putting It All Together

Meal planning, batch cooking, and proper storage are your best friends when it comes to maintaining a healthy, kidney-friendly diet without spending hours in the kitchen every day. By investing some time in planning and preparation, you can enjoy nutritious, delicious meals all week long.

- Weekly Meal Plans: Take the time to plan your meals for the week. This helps you stay organized, ensures variety, and makes grocery shopping more efficient.

- Batch Cooking: Dedicate a few hours once a week to cook large batches of food. This way, you always have something healthy and ready to eat.
- Storing and Reheating: Store your meals properly to maintain their freshness and reheat them safely to enjoy them at their best.

By incorporating these practices into your routine, you'll find that eating well and managing your time efficiently go hand in hand. You'll not only support your kidney health but also free up time for other important aspects of your life. Happy cooking!

Conclusion

Maintaining a kidney-friendly vegan lifestyle is more than just a diet choice; it's a commitment to nurturing your health and well-being through thoughtful and intentional eating. By focusing on nutrient-rich, plant-based foods, you can support your kidneys while enjoying a diverse array of delicious meals. It's about creating habits that integrate seamlessly into your daily life, making healthy eating both enjoyable and sustainable.

One of the key aspects of this lifestyle is understanding the role of different nutrients and how they impact your kidney health. By paying attention to your intake of protein, phosphorus, potassium, and sodium, you can make informed choices that help manage your condition effectively. Each of these nutrients plays a vital role in your body, and balancing them is crucial for optimal kidney function.

Meal planning and preparation are your allies in this journey. By taking the time to plan your meals weekly, batch cook, and store your dishes properly, you ensure that you always have nutritious options at your fingertips. This not only saves time but also reduces the stress of daily cooking, allowing you to focus on other important aspects of your life.

Hydration is another cornerstone of maintaining kidney health. Incorporating a variety of hydrating beverages like smoothies, juices, and herbal teas into your routine can make staying hydrated enjoyable and beneficial. Remember, the goal is to find what works best for you, considering your lifestyle and preferences.

It's essential to approach this lifestyle with flexibility and a positive mindset.

There will be days when sticking to your meal plan feels challenging, and that's perfectly okay. Allow yourself grace and make adjustments as needed. The key is consistency over time, not perfection every day.

Encouragement and final tips: Embrace the learning process and be patient with yourself. This lifestyle change is a journey, not a destination. Celebrate your progress and small victories along the way. Connect with others who are on a similar path for support and inspiration. Online communities, local support groups, or friends and family can provide valuable encouragement and motivation.

Don't hesitate to experiment with new recipes and flavors. A vegan diet offers a world of culinary possibilities, from vibrant salads and hearty soups to decadent desserts and refreshing beverages. Keep exploring and discovering what you love.

Finally, always listen to your body. Pay attention to how different foods make you feel and adjust your diet accordingly. Your body is your best guide in this journey toward better health.

www.ingramcontent.com/pod-product-compliance
Lightning Source LLC
Chambersburg PA
CBHW071832210526
45479CB00001B/99